Breville Smart Air Fryer Oven Cookbook

The Best Quick, Easy and Delicious Air Fryer Oven Recipes for Healthy Meals

Christina Chlebowski

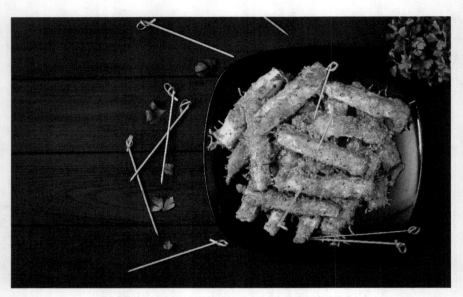

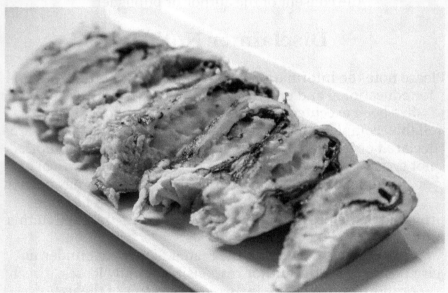

Table of Contents

INTRODUCTION 8

ABOUT THIS ITEM.. 9

WHY BREVILLE IS THE BEST AIR FRYER OVEN 10

HOW DO I USE MY BREVILLE SMART AIR FRYER OVEN 12

HOW TO PREPARE THE OVEN.. 12

ELEMENT IQ 13

BREVILLE SMART VEN AND SMART OVEN PRO COMPARISON

....16

HOW TO CLEAN A BREVILLE SMART AIR FRYER EASILY............. 18

THE OUTER BODY AND DOOR CLEANING 19

CLEANING THE INTERIOR.. 19

WASHING THE CRUMB TRAY.. 19

WASHING OF THE WIRE RACK, BROILING RACK, THE ROASTING PAN, AND THE

PIZZA PAN.. 20

STORAGE.. 20

BREAKFAST RECIPES.. 22

1. SWEET BREAKFAST CASSEROLE....................................... 22

2. AIR FRIED FRENCH TOAST...25

3. WHEAT &SEED BREAD 27

4. CRISPY HAM EGG CUPS 29

5. OLIVES AND KALE 31

6.   STUFFED POBLANOS 32

7.   RASPBERRIES OATMEAL 34

8.   BELL PEPPER EGGS 35

9.   AIR FRYER BREAKFAST FRITTATA 37

10. APPLE-CINNAMON EMPANADAS 38

LAUNCH RECIPES 42

11. HERB-ROASTED TURKEY BREAST 42

12. CRISP CHICKEN CASSEROLE 45

13. FRIED WHOLE CHICKEN 47

14. BARBECUE AIR FRIED CHICKEN 49

15. CORIANDER POTATOES 51

16. ROASTED GARLIC 52

17. AIR FRYER BEEF STEAK 54

18. MUSHROOM MEATLOAF 55

19. SPANISH CHICKEN BAKE 57

20. AIR FRYER MARINATED SALMON 59

21. COCONUT SHRIMP WITH DIP 61

22. AIR FRYER FISH 64

23. LOBSTER TAILS 66

24. CORIANDER ARTICHOKES 68

DINNER RECIPES 70

25. SESAME MUSTARD GREENS 70

26. KALE AND BRUSSELS SPROUTS 72

27. BROCCOLI AND TOMATO SAUCE 73

28. HERBED CARROTS 74

29. CURRIED EGGPLANT 76

APPETIZERS AND SIDE DISHES RECIPES **78**

30. BUTTERED CORN 78

31. BREAD STICKS 80

32. POLENTA STICKS 82

SEA FOOD RECIPES **84**

33. TASTY AIR FRIED COD 84

34. DELICIOUS CATFISH 86

POULTRY RECIPES **88**

35. CREAMY COCONUT CHICKEN 88

36. CHINESE CHICKEN WINGS 89

BEEF AND PORK RECIPES **90**

37. BEEF CURRY 90

38. BEEF AND CABBAGE MIX 92

VEGETABLE RECIPES **94**

39. BALSAMIC ARTICHOKES 94

40. CHEESY ARTICHOKES 96

CONCLUSION **98**

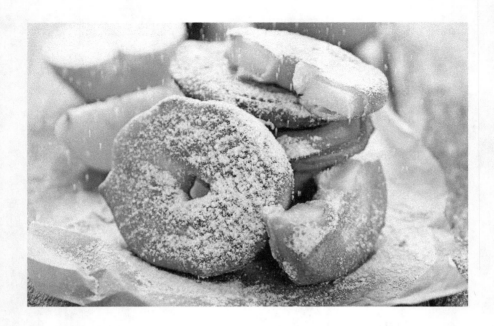

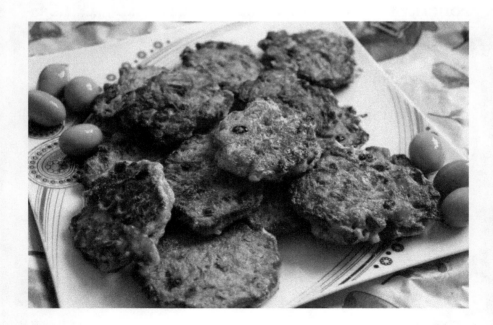

Introduction

Many people enjoy fried food all over the world and would do anything to get their fingers on it. Folks who despise to cook still manage to fry such foods out of their freezer quickly and satisfy their taste buds. However, it is no secret that such fried foods bring a host of health-related problems due to the abundant quantities of oil they soak in while frying. You may use an air fryer to please your taste buds with fried foods without the health- related side effects.

An air-fryer is a modern kitchen device used for cooking food instead of using oil by blowing sweltering air around it. It provides a low-fat variant of foods typically fried in a deep fryer. As a result, unhealthy foods such as French fries, onion rings, and fresh chicken are usually prepared without any oil or up to 80% less fat than conventional cooking techniques.

The Air Fryer offers fried foods and meals that are healthier, allowing you to get rid of the carbs that come from fried foods while still offering you the crunchiness, taste, and consistency you like. By blowing sweltering air (up to 400 ° F) uniformly and rapidly around a food ingredient that is put in a confined environment, this is how the household appliance works. The temperature makes the food part on the outside crispy and dry, but it is soft and moist inside it. You can use an air fryer on pretty much anything. You can barbecue, bake, and roast in addition to frying. The selection of cooking alternatives makes it easier to prepare any meal at any time of the day.

Many modern full-size and already built Air Fryer Toaster Ovens come with an air fryer option these days, but here's a simple truth: many people don't utilize their ovens' air fryer feature. You may ask why? Just because they don't know how to use it.

With that being said, you would need to recognize that unique and innovative kitchen appliances are air fryers that cook your food utilizing hot air circulation. A unique technology named rapid air technology is used for these tolls. And as such, on the inside and perfectly fried on the outside, all the food you cook in these fryers is scrumptious. The next thing you'll notice about air fryers is that they make it possible for you to grill, bake, steam, and roast almost everything you can picture.

Last but not least, you would know that air fryers allow you to cook your foods in a much healthy manner. So many people around the world have just fallen in love with this beautiful and great instrument, and now it's your chance to be one of them.

For the cooks that want a countertop oven that can roast for big meetings, air-fry crispy French fries & family favourites, and dehydrate a wide variety of healthy foods, with the Breville Smart Oven Air with Element IQ. With incredible crispness, the super convection setting cuts cooking time by 30 to 40 per cent. The smart Oven Airspeed heat exchange fan (Super & regular) provides greater cooking power. To ensure that a quick and even heat distribution, super convection produces a greater air volume, suitable for air frying, dehydration, and roasting.

This book includes recipes for air-fried food that will make your jaw drop. Without any remorse, you can find that you can eat French fries and any other fried food. There are

recipes in the book for desserts too! The recipes shared here are going to leave you wanting more. So, let's start cooking without any further delay.

About this item

With air frying features, the Breville Smart Oven Air is much more than a toaster oven. It can also cook slowly, dehydrate, and cook for convection. "TechGearLab (a technology blog) describes it as" one of the few toaster ovens that is a more flexible and reliable tool than most traditional ovens. "If you don't wish to use the considerable big sized oven and wait for it to preheat, the Smart Oven Air certainly has the potential to substitute a conventional oven for most day-to-day uses. If you have the proper and right equipment, you can use it to cook smaller meals and side dishes, make toast, fry good sized batches of food, reheat leftovers, roast a whole chicken, or slow cook. I'm saying that you can practically do a lot of stuff with the Breville Smart Oven Air.

At the right time and when properly tuned to taste, Element IQ delivers the right strength. Nine functions are currently available: toast, bagel, bake, roast, broil, pizza, cookies, reheat, and heat. Voltage ranges between 110 Volts to 120 Volts.

1800 Watts with five heating elements in quartz. Capacity to take six toaster slices, 13- inch pizza. Voltage ranges between 110 volts to 120 Volts Backlit, quick to read LCD moveswhile cooking from blue to orange

Limited Product Warranty for one year

Exterior Dimensions: Width of 15¾ inches by Depth of 18½ inches by Height of11 inches; Interior Dimensions: Width of 13¼ by Depth of 11¼ inches by Height of 5¼ inches; It weighs about 22 pounds

Place the Breville smart oven on a dry, level surface. Ensure that the gap on both sides ofthe appliance is at least 4 inches (10 centimetres) apart.

Why Breville is the Best Air Fryer Oven

- The Smart Oven Air does its functions well, aside from the obvious fact that it is incredibly flexible. The analysis goes into detail about the numerous meals they could make effectively with the unit, including scratch pizza and a slow-cooked stew.
- Chelsea Miller from Foodal (A food Blog) says that she was satisfied after six weeks of Using, and the Smart Oven Air is currently her go-to toasting and baking machine.
- If air frying is not the main feature you are looking for, this is a decent air fryer option because, frankly, there are better options than just air fry. But it is those other features that make the Smart Oven Air a favourite of the public.
- It's a considerable big size toaster oven, able to accommodate up to a 14-pound turkey. To take full advantage of the slow cooking function, there's also space for aDutch oven.
- The device is good at heating meals to the right

temperatures because of the convection technology when getting them to the ideal texture. Your fries would be crispy from the outside and fluffy from the inside.

- To help make your work easier, the appliance has a simple monitor and 13 preset cooking programs. But before cooking, you may also want to acquaint yourself with the toggle switches and settings to get a feeling of their functions.

How Do I Use My Breville Smart Air Fryer Oven

The Breville Smart Oven Appliance comes with a Power supply cord short in length to reduce or minimize kitchen hazards or property damage from tripping, pulling, or getting entangled with another longer cord.

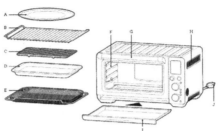

Source: Breville Smart Oven Air Instruction Manual
A is a Pizza Pan (Non-Stick)
B is a Wire Rack that is reversible for
Eight separate Rack Positions C is 9
inches by 13 Inches Broiling Rack
D is 9 inches by 13 Inches Roasting Pan
E is the Air Fry Basket, also
called the Dehydrate Basket
F is the Light for the Oven
G is the Door Handle

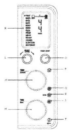

Source: Breville Smart Oven Air Instruction Manual
How to Prepare the Oven
It is essential to operate the oven empty for 20 minutes to remove any protective substances from the heating elements. Ensure that the room is adequately ventilated, as the oven can produce vapours. These vapours are harmless and are not harmful to the oven's efficiency.

Remove all packaging material, marketing labels, and tape from the oven and securely discard them.

Remove the polyfoam packing from the crumb tray, wire shelves, broiling rack, roasting pan, air fry / dehydrate basket, and pizza pan. Wash them in wet, soapy water with a soft sponge and then clean and dry thoroughly. Wipe a smooth, damp sponge around the inside of the oven. Thoroughly Dry.

Put the oven on a dry, level surface. Ensure that the minimum space gap is 4 inches (10 centimetres) on both sides of the machine and 6 inches (15 centimetres) above the machine.

In the oven, insert the crumb plate.

Fully unwind the power cord and put the power plug into a rooted power outlet.

The oven alarm will whistle, and it will illuminate the LCD panel. The options for the feature are shown with the Toast settings indicator.

Switch the Confirm dial selector to the right till the indicator instructs the PIZZA feature. Click the button for Pick or Pause. Red will illuminate the button backlight, orange will illuminate the LCD panel, and the oven alarm will sound.

A blinking 'PREHEATING' will show the LCD panel. A warning will sound once the oven has ended the preheating cycle.

The timer will be shown, and it will start counting down automatically.

The oven alarm will sound at the end of the cooking cycle, the backlight of the START or STOP button will go out, and the LCD panel will illuminate white.

The oven is ready for use now.

Element IQ

Element IQ, a kitchen technology that changes the heating elements' power to cook food more evenly and quickly, is featured in the Breville Smart Oven Air. With our recommended configuration, each of the oven's functions is preset. That being said, depending on the recipe quantity and your taste, we suggest playing with these.

Your custom setting will stay in the oven's memory until you adjust or reset the oven to the original factory setting, even if the power cord is uninstalled. The FROZEN and TEMPERATURE CONVERSION buttons are pressed and held together for 5 seconds to do this.

Operating Your Breville Oven

1.   In the desired rack location, insert the wire rack. On the left-hand side of the oven door window, the rack positions are conveniently published. Four groove positions exist. To allow two rack positions for each groove, the rack can be installed either facing an upward or downward.

2.   Turn the Pick or CONFIRM dial on until the indicator on the LCD panel reaches the desired setting.

3.   For the chosen setting, the top figure on the LCD screen clearly shows the preset cooking temperature. It shows the level of darkness for the TOAST and BAGEL settings. To decrease the temperature or to the right to raise the temperature, turn the TEMPERATURE dial to the left.

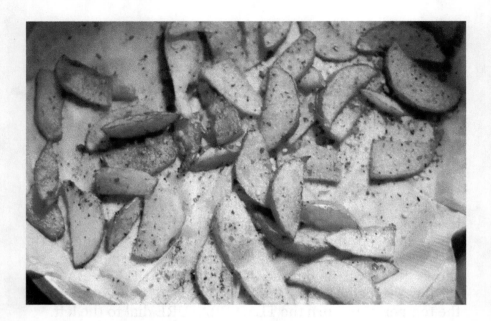

Breville Smart ven and Smart Oven Pro Comparison

In its full-size Smart Oven line, Breville offers three models: The Smart Oven, the Smart Oven Plus, and the Smart Oven Pro. They have the same measurements, and the design and cooking technology are present in each model. A slow cooking feature is added to the Smart Oven Plus that allows you to cook for up to 10 hours before switching to a warm mode automatically. The slow cooking feature, an internal oven light, is included in the Smart Oven Pro.

For $249.99, the Smart Oven is available for purchase online on Amazon and numerous other outlets. The smart Oven Plus goes for 249.95 dollars. And, from Amazon and other outlets, the Smart Oven Pro is $269.95.

For more accessible access to the built-in smart features, the Smart Oven Pro comes with an LCD screen display, allowing you to select ten cooking functions with 6-slice toaster power, a 13-inch pizza, and space roast a whole chicken, or a 9-cup muffin tray. The Element IQ technology transfers the power across the oven with the Smart Oven Pro to deliver accurate cooking temperatures required for perfect results throughout the ten preset cooking features. It contains all nine of the other Smart Oven features with one additional feature like a slow cooker. This allows you to cook a whole chicken well enough without drying it out or compromising the interior's temperature consistency. It cooks at 1800 watts, making it an efficient heat mover, and comes with four separate accessories (two enamel pans, a pizza pan, and an oven rack). It appears in different materials like stainless, black, and cherry red (three distinct classic kitchen colours). It uses a classic toaster oven configuration with Breville's Smart Element IQ to spread heat equally and avoid over or under-cooking. To expel cold air and bring up hot air needed even for cooking, a powerful fan transfers air quickly. It has a bright LED that displays all your choices and settings and an emergency stop shut-off.

Who It's For: Cooks that do not want to put on their big oven but still need an array of services that is similar to a more significant appliance (especially in warm and temperateclimates).

Pros:

- Ten different features of cooking
- Includes choice for slow cooking
- Three classic colours for the kitchen
- A happy medium between heating and capacity is reached by small to medium-sized
- Res

tricted

warranty

for   one

yearCons:

- Over time, LEDs can cloud
- It gets scorching on the appliance's exterior walls
- The ventilator can be loud,
- The toast feature is terrible,

The 23 Liters size of the Smart Oven Air Fryer makes room for 1 kilogram of French friestoast about six slices of bread, with the ability to roast a whole chicken, slow cooking witha 4.2 Liter Dutch oven and 13 inches or 30-centimetre pizza and 9 cup muffin trays suit it comfortably. For several different cooking techniques, smart algorithms direct power to where and when required to establish the optimal cooking environment. It removes cold spots for accurate and even cooking through sensors and digital PID temperature control. The guesswork is taken out of cooking by individual heating elements andsuitable rack locations. The device comes in two distinct classic kitchen colours and includes a non-stick interior, which is much easier to clean and prevents staining. The Element IQ of Breville transfers heat around more effectively, each time giving you a better result. It has a brightly illuminated LED, plus dial control knobs, that gives you allyour functions and choices. The automatic shutdown mechanism prevents the oven fromgoing past the cooking stage and is a useful safety feature.

Who It's For: Cooks with a budget that is the final

determining factor or who do not needthe slow cook feature.
Pros:

- Three cooking accessories come along with it
- Nine tasks, which include baking,
- Two classic colours for the kitchen
- Oven balances, small to medium scale, heating time with the capability
- Res

tricted
warranty
for   one
yearCons:

- Fuse issues can occur sooner than expected,
- With time, the display appears to become cloudy
- Over time, enamel pans may form small cracks.
- No slow choice for cooking
- It also has an internal light that, when the cooking is finished, automatically turnson.

An outstanding oven that worked well across the board is the Breville Smart Oven Plus (and the other line) models. It provides ample food power to make your full-sized home oven a viable replacement.

There are some decent looking appliances made by Breville, and these are no exception. They feel solid and have a stunning look that almost complements any kitchen décor. If you wouldn't want to put on your oven and heat your whole house to make a pizza, we suggest using a convection toaster. They're incredibly helpful when you're cooking for onenight, and you need a little bit of flexibility to build your whole meal. It's simpler, faster, and probably easier to maintain than your big oven. Given the time you might spend making up new dishes for yourself, your friends, and family, that's an advantage on its own.

How to Clean a Breville Smart Air Fryer Easily

Take precautions to observe that the oven is switched off by pulling out the power plug from the electrical outlet before cleaning.

The outer body and door cleaning

With a smooth, damp sponge, wash the outer body. To prevent the build-up of stains, a non-abrasive liquid cleanser or mild spray solution can be used. Until washing, add the cleanser to the sponge and not to the oven body.

Using a glass cleaner or pleasant detergent and a soft, wet sponge or soft plastic scouring pad to clean the glass door. As these can scrape the oven body, you should not use an abrasive cleanser or metal scouring pad.

Wipe a smooth, damp cloth on the LCD display screen. Add the cleanser and not the surface of the LCD to the fabric. It can scratch the surface by wiping with a dry cloth or abrasive cleaners.

Before putting or plugging in the power plug into an electrical outlet and switching the oven, let all surfaces dry correctly.

Cleaning the interior

The walls inside the oven have a non - stick surface for quick cleaning. Wipe the walls with a smooth, damp sponge to wash any splattering that can occur when cooking. To preventthe build-up of stains, a non-abrasive liquid cleanser or mild spray solution can be used. Until washing, add the cleanser to the sponge, not to the surface of the oven. Stop hittingthe heating elements of quartz.

Washing the crumb tray

Drag the crumb tray out after each usage and remove the crumbs. Clean the tray with a smooth, damp sponge. To prevent the build-up of stains, a non-abrasive liquid cleaner can be used. Until washing, add the cleanser to the sponge, not to the plate. Properly Dry. Dip the tray into warm and soapy water then wipe with a soft sponge or soft plastic scouring pad to remove the grease from baking. Properly rinse it, then dry it.

Following cleaning and before putting the power plug into a power outlet and turning the oven on, always reinsert the crumb tray into the oven.

Washing of the Wire Rack, Broiling rack, the Roasting Pan, and the Pizza Pan.

Wash all of the accessories with a soft sponge or soft plastic scouring pad in warm soapy water. Rinse and thoroughly dry. To clean any of the accessories, do not use abrasive cleansers, metal scouring pads, or metal utensils to harm the surfaces.

We do not recommend sticking these in the dishwasher to prolong the life of your accessories.

Storage

Ensure that by pulling out the power plug from the electrical socket, the oven is switchedoff.

Before disassembling and cleaning, make the oven and all accessories fully to cool off. Ensure that the oven is completely dry as well as all other accessories.

Ensure that the crumb tray is placed into the oven; place the broiling rack in the roasting pan and place it at the middle rack height location on the wire rack.

Ensure that the door is locked.

Keep the appliance on its support legs in an upright position, standing level. Do not store the top with something. The only exception is the optional Serving Tray and Breville Bamboo Cutting Board.

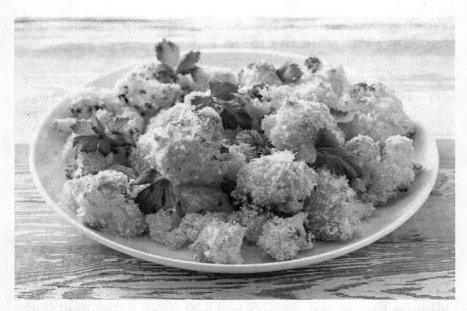

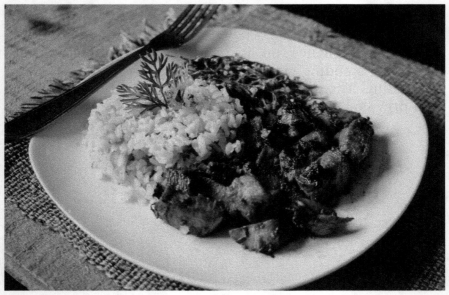

Breakfast Recipes

1. Sweet Breakfast Casserole

- Three tablespoons brown sugar

- Four tablespoons margarine

- Two tablespoons white sugar

- 1/2 tsp. cinnamon powder

- 1/2 cup flour

- For the casserole:

- Two eggs

- Two tablespoons white sugar

- 2 and 1/2 cups white flour

- 1 tsp. baking soda

- 1 tsp. baking powder

- Two eggs

- 1/2 cup milk

- 2 cups margarine milk

- Four tablespoons margarine

- Zest from 1 lemon, grated

- 1 and 2/3 cup blueberries

Directions:

In a bowl, mix eggs with two tablespoons white sugar, 2 and 1/2 cups white flour, baking powder, baking soda, two eggs, milk, margarine milk, four tablespoons margarine, lemonzest, and blueberries, mix it and pour it into a pan that can enter your air fryer.

In other bowls, mix three tablespoons brown sugar

with two tablespoons white sugar, four tablespoons margarine, 1/2 cup of flour, and cinnamon, mix it until you obtain a crumble and spread over blueberries mix.

Place in the preheated air fryer and bake at 300 °F for 30 minutes. Divide among plates and serve for breakfast.

2. Air Fried French Toast

- Two slices of sourdough bread

- Three eggs

- One tablespoon of margarine

- 1 tsp. of liquid vanilla

- Three tsp.s of honey

- Two tablespoons of Greek yoghurt Berries

Directions:

Preheat the air fryer to 356°F.

Pour the vanilla into the eggs and whisk to mix.

Spread the margarine on all sides of the bread and

soak in the eggs to absorb.

Place it in the deep fryer basket and cook for 3

minutes. Turn the bread over and cook for another

3 minutes.

Transfer to a place, top with yoghurt and berries

with a sprinkle of honey.

3. Wheat &Seed Bread

- 31/2 ounces of flour

- 1 tsp. of yeast

- 1 tsp. of salt

- Three &1/2 ounces of wheat flour ¼ cup of pumpkin seeds

Directions:

Mix the wheat flour, yeast, salt, seeds and the plain flour in a large bowl. Stir in ¾ cup of lukewarm water and keep stirring until dough becomes soft.

Knead for another 5 minutes until the dough becomes elastic and smooth.

Mould into a ball and cover with a plastic bag. Set aside for 30 minutes for it to rise. Heat your air fryer to 392°F.

Transfer the dough into a small pizza pan and place in the air fryer. Bake for 18 minutes until golden. Remove the dough and then place it on a wire rack to cool.

4. Crispy Ham Egg Cups

- Four large eggs.

- 4: 1-oz. slices deli ham

- ½ cup shredded medium Cheddar cheese.

- ¼ cup diced green bell pepper.

- 2 tbsp. diced red bell pepper.

- 2 tbsp. diced white onion.

- 2 tbsp. Full-fat sour cream.

Directions:

On top of four baking cups, put the ham there.

Take a big bowl, and with sour cream, mix the eggs. With green pepper, onion and red pepper mix the ham with it.

Pour into a ham-lined baking cups. Top with

Cheddar. Place cups into the air fryer basket. Adjust the temperature to 320 Degrees F and set the timer for 12 minutes or until the tops are browned. Serve warm.

5. Olives and Kale

- Four eggs; whisked One cup kale; chopped.

- ½ cup black olives, pitted and sliced

- 2 tbsp. cheddar; grated

- Cooking spray A pinch of salt

Directions:

Take a bowl and mix the eggs with the rest of the ingredients except the cooking spray and whisk well.

Now, take a pan that fits in your air fryer and grease it with the cooking spray, pour the olives mixture inside, spread Put the pan into the machine and cook at 360°F for 20 minutes. Serve for breakfast hot.

6. **Stuffed Poblanos**

- ½ lb. spicy ground pork breakfast sausage

- Four large poblano peppers

- Four large eggs.

- ½ cup full-fat sour cream.

- 4 oz. Full-fat softened cream cheese.

- ¼ canned sliced tomatoes as well as green chiles.

- 8 tbsp. shredded pepper jack cheese

Directions:

Crumble and brown the ground sausage in a medium skillet over medium heat, until there is no pink remaining. Remove it out of the pan and drain the fat. Beat the eggs in the pan, scatter and cook until they don't run anymore.

Place cooked sausage in a large bowl and fold in cream cheese. Mix in diced tomatoes and chiles.

Gently fold in eggs

Cut a 4"–5" slit in the top of each poblano, removing the seeds and white membrane with a small knife. Separate the filling into four and spoon carefully into each pepper. Top each with 2 tbsp— pepper jack cheese.

Inside the air fryer basket put each petter. Adjust the temperature to 350 Degrees F and set the timer for 15 minutes.The pepper would be brown and would be soft when it is ready. Serve it with sour cream and enjoy your meal.

7. **Raspberries Oatmeal**

- 1 ½ cups coconut; shredded

- ½ cups raspberries

- Two cups almond milk

- ¼ tsp. nutmeg, ground

- 2 tsp. Stevia

- ½ tsp. cinnamon powder

- Cooking spray

Directions:

Grease the air fryer's pan with cooking spray, mix all the ingredients inside, cover and cook at 360°F for 15 minutes. Divide into bowls and serve.

8. Bell Pepper Eggs

- Four medium green bell peppers

- ¼ medium onion; peeled and chopped

- 3 oz. cooked ham; chopped

- Eight large eggs.

- 1 cup mild Cheddar cheese

Directions:

The top of each bell pepper should be removed.

With a small knife remove the seeds as well and the

white membranes. Place ham and onion into each

pepper.

Crack two eggs into each pepper. Top with ¼ cup

cheese per pepper. Place into the airfryer basket

Set the timer for 15 minutes and change the temperature to 360 degrees Fahrenheit. When fully cooked, peppers will be tender, and eggs will be firm. Serve immediately.

9. **Air Fryer Breakfast Frittata**

- ¼ pound breakfast sausage fully cooked and crumbled Four eggs, lightly beaten

- ½ cup Monterey Jack cheese, shredded

- Two tablespoons red bell pepper, diced

- One green onion, chopped

- One pinch cayenne pepper

Directions:

Preheat the Air fryer to 3650F and grease a non-stick 6x2-inch cake pan.Whisk together eggs with sausage, green onion, bell pepper, cheese and cayenne in a bowl. Transfer the egg mixture in the prepared cake pan and place in the air fryer.

Cook for about 20 minutes and serve warm.

10.   **Apple-Cinnamon Empanadas**

- 2-3 baking apples, peeled & diced

- Two tsp.s of cinnamon

- 1/4 cup white sugar

- One tablespoon brown sugar

- One tablespoon of water

- 1/2 tablespoon cornstarch

- ¼ tsp. of vanilla extract

- Two tablespoons of margarine or margarine

- Four pre-made empanada dough shells (Goya)

Directions:

In a bowl, add together white sugar, brown sugar, cornstarch and cinnamon; set aside. Put the diced apples in a pot and place on a stovetop.

Add the combined dry ingredients to the apples, then add the water, vanilla extract, and margarine; stirring well to mix.

Cover pot and cook on high heat. Once it starts boiling, lower heat and simmers until the apples are soft, removes from the heat and cold.

Lay the empanada shells on a clean counter. Spoon the mixture of apple and put it inside each of the shells, being careful to prevent spillage over the edges. Fold shells to cover apple mixture fully, seal edges with water, pressing down to secure with a fork.

With tin foil, cover the basket of the air fryer, but

leave the edges uncovered so that air can circulate through the basket. Place the empanadas shells in the foil-lined air fryer basket, set temperature at 350°F and timer for 15 minutes.

Slide the frying basket out halfway through and turn the empanadas with the use of a spatula. When golden in colour, extract and serve on plates directly from the basket.

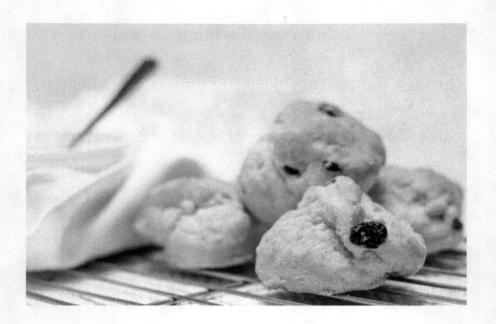

Launch Recipes

11. Herb-Roasted Turkey Breast

- 3 lb turkey breast

- Rub Ingredients:

- 2 tbsp olive oil

- 2 tbsp lemon juice

- 1 tbsp minced Garlic

- 2 tsp ground mustard

- 2 tsp kosher salt

- 1 tsp pepper

- 1 tsp dried rosemary

- 1 tsp dried thyme

- 1 tsp ground sage

Directions:

Take a small bowl and thoroughly combine the Rub Ingredients: in it. Rub this on the outside of the turkey breast and under any loose skin.

Place the coated turkey breast keeping skin side up on a cooking tray.

Below the cooking chamber of the Air Fryer put the drip pan. Select Air Fry option, post this, adjust the temperature to 360°F and the time to one hour, then touch start.

When preheated, add the food to the cooking tray in the lowest position.

Close the lid for cooking.

When the Air Fry program is complete, check to make sure that the thickest portion of the meat reads at least 160°F, remove the turkey and let it rest for 10 minutes before slicing and serving.

12. Crisp Chicken Casserole

- 3 cup chicken, shredded

- 12 oz bag egg noodles

- 1/2 large onion

- 1/2 cup chopped carrots

- 1/4 cup frozen peas

- 1/4 cup frozen broccoli pieces

- Two stalks celery chopped

- 5 cup chicken broth

- 1 tsp garlic powder

- salt and pepper to taste

- 1 cup cheddar cheese, shredded

- One package French's onions

- 1/4 cup sour cream

- One can cream of chicken and mushroom soup

Directions:

Place the chicken, vegetables, garlic powder, salt and pepper, and broth and stir. Then place it into the Instant Pot Duo Crisp Air Fryer Basket.

Press or lightly stir the egg noodles into the mix until damp/wet.Select the option Air Fryer and cook for 4 minutes.

Stir in the sour cream, can of soup, cheese, and 1/3 of the French's onions.

Top with the remaining French's onions and close the Air Fryer lid and cook for about ten more minutes.

13. Fried Whole Chicken

- Ingredients:

- 1 Whole chicken

- 2 Tbsp or spray of oil of choice

- 1 tsp garlic powder

- 1 tsp onion powder

- 1 tsp paprika

- 1 tsp Italian seasoning

- 2 Tablespoon of Montreal Steak Seasoning

- 1.5 cup chicken broth

Directions:

Truss and wash the chicken.

Mix the seasoning and rub a little amount on the

chicken. Pour the broth inside the Instant Pot Duo Crisp Air Fryer. The chicken should be put inside the air fryer basket.

Select the option Air Fry and Close the Air Fryer lid and cook for 25 minutes.

Rub the top of the chicken with oil or spray it and rub it with a quarter the seasoning. Close the air fryer lid and for 10 minutes air fry again at 400°F.

Flip the chicken, spray it with oil, and rub with the remaining seasoning.

Again air fries it for another ten minutes.

Allow the chicken to rest for 10 minutes.

14.Barbecue Air Fried Chicken

- One teaspoon Liquid Smoke

- Two cloves Fresh Garlic smashed

- 1/2 cup Apple Cider Vinegar

- 3 pounds Chuck Roast well-marbled with intramuscular fat

- 1 Tablespoon Kosher Salt

- 1 Tablespoon Freshly Ground Black Pepper

- Two teaspoons Garlic Powder

- 1.5 cups Barbecue Sauce

- 1/4 cup Light Brown Sugar + more for sprinkling

- 2 Tablespoons honey optional and in place of 2 TBL sugar

Directions:

Add meat to the Instant Pot Duo Crisp Air Fryer Basket, spreading out the meat. Select the option, Air Fry.

Close the Air Fryer lid and cook at 300 degrees F for 8 minutes. Pause the Air Fryer andflip the meat over after 4 minutes.

Remove the lid and baste with more barbecue sauce and sprinkle with a little brown sugar. Again Close the Air Fryer lid and set the temperature at 400°F for 9 minutes.

Watch meat though the lid and flip it over after 5 minutes.

15. Coriander Potatoes

- 1 pound gold potatoes, peeled and cut into wedges Salt and black pepper to the taste

- One tablespoon tomato sauce

- Two tablespoons coriander, chopped

- ½ teaspoon garlic powder

- One teaspoon chilli powder

- One tablespoon olive oil

Directions:

In a bowl, put both the potatoes with the tomato sauce and the other ingredients, toss, and transfer to the air fryer's basket. Cook for 25 minutes at 370 degrees F, divide between plates and serve as a side dish.

16. Roasted Garlic

- One medium head garlic

- 2 tsp. avocado oil

Directions:

Remove any hanging excess peel from the garlic but leave the cloves covered. Cut off ¼

of the head of garlic, exposing the tips of the cloves

Drizzle with avocado oil. Place the garlic head into a small sheet of aluminium foil, completely enclosing it. Place it in the basket of an air fryer.

Change the temperature and set the timer to 400 degrees F for 20 minutes. If the head of your garlic is slightly smaller, check it after 15 minutes.

Garlic should be golden brown when finished and

very soft when finished.

Cloves should pop out to serve and be spread or sliced quickly. It can be preserved in the refrigerator in an airtight container.

You may also freeze individual cloves on a baking sheet, then store together in a freezer-safe storage bag once frozen.

17. **Air Fryer Beef Steak**

- 1 tbsp. Olive oil

- Pepper and salt

- 2 pounds of ribeye steak

Directions:

Preparing the ingredients. Season the meat with pepper and salt. Preheat instant, crisp air fryer to 356 degrees and spritz with olive oil. Air frying. Close air fryer lid. Set temperature to 356°f, and set time to 7 minutes. Cook steak 7 minutes. Flip and cook an additional 6 minutes. Let the meat sit 2-5 minutes to rest. Slice and serve with salad.

18.Mushroom Meatloaf

- 14-ounce lean ground beef

- One chorizo sausage, chopped finely

- One small onion, chopped

- One garlic clove, minced

- Two tablespoons fresh cilantro, chopped

- Three tablespoons breadcrumbs

- One egg

- Salt and ground black pepper

- Two tablespoons fresh mushrooms sliced thinly

- Three tablespoons olive oil

Directions:

Preparing the ingredients. Preheat the instant, crisp

air fryer to 390 degrees f.

In a big-sized bowl, put all ingredients except mushrooms and mix till well combined.

In a baking pan, place the beef mixture.

Use the back of a spatula to smooth the surface.

Top with mushroom slices and gently, press into the meatloaf.Drizzle with oil evenly.

Air frying. Arrange the pan in the instant, crisp air fryer basket, close air fryer lid and cook for about 25 minutes.

Cut the meatloaf in desires size wedges and serve.

19.Spanish Chicken Bake

- ½ onion, quartered

- ½ red onion, quartered

- ½ lb. potatoes, quartered

- Four garlic cloves

- Four tomatoes, quartered

- 1/8 cup chorizo

- ¼ teaspoon paprika powder

- Four chicken thighs, boneless

- ¼ teaspoon dried oregano

- ½ green bell pepper, julienned

- Salt Black pepper

Directions:

Toss chicken, veggies, and all the Ingredients: in a

baking tray.

Press "Power Button" of Air Fry Oven and turn the dial to select the "Bake" Mode. Press the Time button and again turn the dial to set the cooking time to 25 minutes. Now push the Temp button and rotate the dial to set the temperature at 425 degrees F. Once preheated, place the baking pan inside and close its lid.

Serve warm.

20.   **Air Fryer Marinated Salmon**

- Four salmon fillets or one 1lb fillet cut into four pieces

- 1 Tbsp brown sugar

- ½ Tbsp Minced Garlic

- 6 Tbsps Soy Sauce

- ¼ cup Dijon Mustard

- 1 Green onion finely chopped

Directions:

Take a bowl and whisk together soy sauce, dijon mustard, brown sugar, and minced garlic. Pour this mixture over salmon fillets, making sure that all the fillets are covered. Refrigerate and marinate for 20-30 minutes.

Remove salmon fillets from marinade and place them in greased or lined on the tray in the Instant Pot Duo Crisp Air Fryer basket, close the lid.

Select the Air Fry option and Air Fry for around 12 minutes at 400°F.

Remove from Instant Pot Duo Crisp Air Fryer and top with chopped green onions.

21. Coconut Shrimp with Dip

- 1 lb raw shrimp that is peeled and deveined with tail on

- Two eggs are beaten

- ¼ cup Panko Breadcrumbs

- 1 tsp salt

- ¼ tsp black pepper

- ½ cup All-Purpose Flour

- ½ cup unsweetened shredded coconut

- Oil for spraying

Directions:

Clean and dry the shrimp. Set it aside.

Take three bowls. Put flour in the first bowl. Beat

eggs in the second bowl. Mix coconut, breadcrumbs, salt, and black pepper in the third bowl.

Select the Air Fry option and adjust the temperature to 390°F. Push start, and preheating will start.

Dip each shrimp in flour followed by the egg and then coconut mixture, ensuring shrimp is covered on all sides during each dip.

Once the preheating is done, place shrimp in a single layer on a greased tray in the basket of the Instant Pot Duo Crisp Air Fryer.

Spray the shrimp with oil lightly, and then close the Air Fryer basket lid.

Cook for around 4 minutes.

After 4 minutes open the Air Fryer basket lid and flip the shrimp over. Respray the shrimp with oil, close the Air Fryer basket lid, and cook for five more minutes.

Remove shrimp from the basket and serve with Thai Sweet Chili Sauce.

22.   **Air Fryer Fish**

- 4-6 Whiting Fish fillets cut in half

- Oil to mist

- Fish Seasoning

- ¾ cup very fine cornmeal

- ¼ cup flour

- 2 tsp old bay

- 1 ½ tsp salt

- 1 tsp paprika

- ½ tsp garlic powder

- ½ tsp black pepper

Directions:

Put the Ingredients: for fish seasoning in a Ziplock

bag and shake it well. Set aside. Rinse the fish

fillets with paper towels and pat them dry. Make sure they're still damp. In a ziplock container, put the fish fillets and shake until they are fully coated with seasoning.

To allow any excess flour to fall off, position the fillets on a baking rack.Grease the bottom of the Instant Pot Duo Crisp Air Fryer basket tray and place the fillets on the tray. Close the lid, select the Air Fry option and cook filets on 400°F for 10 minutes. Open the Air Fryer lid and spray the fish with oil on the side facing up before flipping it over, ensure that the fish is fully coated. Flip and cook another side of the fish for 7 minutes. Remove the fish and serve.

23.   **Lobster Tails**

- Two 6oz lobster tails

- 1 tsp salt

- 1 tsp chopped chives

- 2 Tbsp unsalted butter melted

- 1 Tbsp minced garlic

- 1 tsp lemon juice

Directions:

Combine butter, garlic, salt, chives, and lemon juice to prepare butter mixture.

Butterfly lobster tails by cutting through shell followed by removing the meat and resting it on top of the shell.

Place them on the tray in the Instant Pot Duo

Crisp Air Fryer basket and spread butter over the top of lobster meat. Close the Air Fryer lid, select the

Air Fry option and cook on 380°F for 4 minutes.

Open the Air Fryer lid and spread more butter on top, cook for extra 2-4 minutes untildone.

24.   **Coriander Artichokes**

- 12 oz. artichoke hearts

- 1 tbsp. lemon juice

- 1 tsp. Coriander, ground

- ½ tsp. Cumin seeds

- ½ tsp. olive oil

- Salt and black pepper to taste.

Directions:

Combine all the ingredients in the foreign pan that suits your air fryer, toss, place the pan in the fryer and cook for 15 minutes at 370 ° F.

Divide the mix between plates and serve as a side dish.

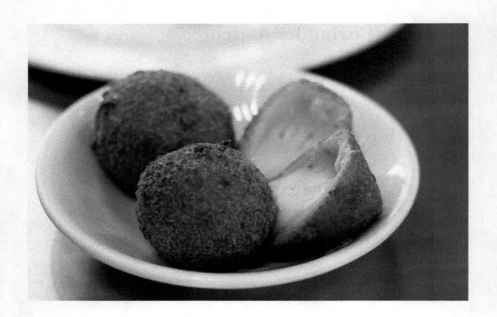

Dinner Recipes

25.   Sesame Mustard Greens

- Two garlic cloves, minced

- 1 pound mustard greens, torn

- One tablespoon olive oil

- ½ cup yellow onion, sliced

- Salt and black pepper to the taste

- Three tablespoons veggie stock

- ¼ teaspoon dark sesame oil

Directions:

Heat a pan that fits your air fryer with the oil over medium heat, add onions, stir and brown them for 5 minutes.

Add garlic, stock, greens, salt and pepper, stir,

introduce in your air fryer and cook at 350

°F for 6 minutes.

Add sesame oil, toss to coat, divide among plates

and serve.

26.   Kale and Brussels Sprouts

- 1 lb. Brussels sprouts, trimmed

- 3 oz. mozzarella, shredded

- 2 cups kale, torn

- 1 tbsp. olive oil

- Salt and black pepper to taste.

Directions:

In a pan that fits the air fryer, combine all the Ingredients: except the mozzarella and toss. Cook at 380°F for 15 minutes.

Divide between plates, sprinkle the cheese on top and serve.

27.   **Broccoli and Tomato Sauce**

- One broccoli head, florets separated

- ¼ cup scallions; chopped

- ½ cup tomato sauce

- 1 tbsp. olive oil

- 1 tbsp. sweet paprika

- Salt and black pepper to taste.

Directions:

In a pan that fits the air fryer, combine the broccoli with the rest of the Ingredients: toss. Put the pan in the fryer and cook at 380°F for 15 minutes

Divide between plates and serve.

28.   Herbed Carrots

- Six large carrots, peeled and sliced lengthwise

- Two tablespoons olive oil

- ½ tablespoon fresh oregano, chopped

- ½ tablespoon fresh parsley, chopped

- Salt and black pepper, to taste

- Two tablespoons olive oil, divided

- ½ cup fat-free Italian dressing

- Salt, to taste

Directions:

Preheat the Air fryer to 360-degree F and grease an

Air fryer basket. Mix the carrot slices and olive oil in

a bowl and toss to coat well.

Arrange the carrot slices in the Air fryer basket and

cook for about 12 minutes.

Dish out the carrot slices onto serving plates and sprinkle with herbs, salt and blackpepper.

Transfer into the Air fryer basket and cook for two more minutes. Dish out and serve hot.

29.   **Curried Eggplant**

- One large eggplant, cut into ½-inch thick slices

- One garlic clove, minced

- ½ fresh red chilli, chopped

- One tablespoon vegetable oil

- ¼ teaspoon curry powder

- Salt, to taste

Directions:

Begin with heating your Air Fryer to a temperature of 300 degrees F and grease an Air fryer basket.

Arrange the eggplant slices in the Air fryer basket

and cook for about 10 minutes, tossing once in between.

Dish out onto serving plates and serve hot.

Appetizers and Side Dishes

Recipes

30.   Buttered Corn

- Two corn on the cob

- Salt

- ground black pepper

- Two tablespoons butter, softened and divided

Directions:

Sprinkle the cobs evenly with salt and black pepper.

Then, rub with one tablespoon of butter.

With one piece of foil, wrap each cob.

Press "Power Button" of Air Fry Oven and turn the dial to select the "Air Fry" mode. Press the

Time button and again turn the dial to set the cooking time to 20 minutes. Now push the Temp button and rotate the dial to set the temperature at 320 degrees F. Press the "Start/Pause" button to start.

When the unit beeps to show that it is preheated, open the lid. Arrange the cobs in "Air Fry Basket" and insert in the oven.

Serve warm.

31. Bread Sticks

- One egg 1/8 teaspoon of cinnamon

- A Pinch of ground nutmeg

- A Pinch of ground cloves

- Salt, to taste

- Two bread slices

- One tablespoon butter softened

- Nonstick cooking spray

- One tablespoon icing sugar

Directions:

In a bowl, add the eggs, cinnamon, nutmeg, cloves and salt and beat until well combined. The butter should be spread on both sides of the slices evenly. Cut each bread slice into strips.

Dip bread strips into egg mixture evenly.

Press "Power Button" of Air Fry Oven and turn the dial to select the "Air Fry" mode. Press the Time button and again turn the dial to set the cooking time to 6 minutes. Now push the Temp button and rotate the dial to set the temperature at 355 degrees F. Press the "Start/Pause" button to start.

When the unit beeps to show that it is preheated, open the lid. Arrange the breadsticks in "Air Fry Basket" and insert in the oven.

After 2 minutes of cooking, spray both sides of the bread strips with cooking spray. Serve immediately with the topping of icing sugar.

32.   **Polenta Sticks**

- One tablespoon oil

- 2½ cups cooked polenta

- Salt, to taste

- ¼ cup Parmesan cheese

Directions:

Place the polenta in a lightly greased baking pan.

With a plastic wrap, cover and refrigerate for about 1 hour or until set. Remove from the refrigerator and cut into desired sized slices.

Sprinkle with salt.

Press "Power Button" of Air Fry Oven and turn the dial to select the "Air Fry" mode. Press the

Time button and again turn the dial to set the cooking time to 6 minutes. Now push the Temp button and rotate the dial to set the temperature at 350 degrees F.Press the "Start/Pause" button to start.

When the unit beeps to show that it is preheated, open the lid. Arrange the pan over the "Wire Rack" and insert in the oven. Top with cheese and serve.

Sea Food Recipes

33.   Tasty Air Fried Cod

- Two codfish, 7 ounces each

- A drizzle of sesame oil

- Salt and black pepper to the taste

- 1 cup of water

- One teaspoon dark soy sauce

- Four tablespoons light soy sauce

- One tablespoon sugar

- Three tablespoons olive oil

- Four ginger slices

- Three spring onions, chopped

- Two tablespoons coriander, chopped

Directions:

Season fish with salt, pepper, drizzle sesame oil, rub well and leave aside for 10 minutes. Add fish to your air fryer and cook at 356 degrees F for 12 minutes.

Meanwhile, over medium heat, heat a pot with water, add lighter and darker soy sauce and sugar, stir, bring to boil and remove from the heat.

Heat a pan with the olive oil over medium heat, add ginger and green onions, stir, cook for a few minutes and take off the heat.

Divide fish on plates, top with ginger and green onions, drizzle soy sauce mix, sprinkle coriander and serve right away.

34.   **Delicious Catfish**

- Four catfish fillets

- Salt and black pepper to the taste

- A pinch of sweet paprika

- One tablespoon parsley, chopped

- One tablespoon lemon juice

- One tablespoon olive oil Directions:

Season catfish fillets with salt, pepper, paprika, drizzle oil, rub well, Cook for 20 minutes at 400 degrees F, flipping the fish after 10 minutes.

Divide fish on plates, drizzle lemon juice all over, sprinkle parsley and serve.

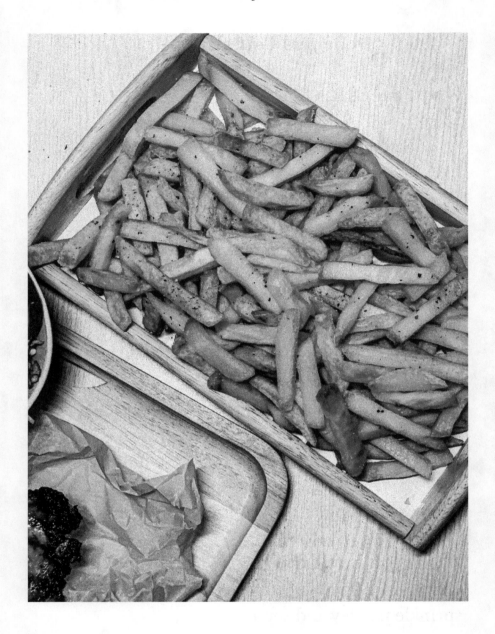

Poultry Recipes

35.　　Creamy Coconut Chicken

- Four big chicken legs

- Five teaspoons turmeric powder

- Two tablespoons ginger, grated

- Salt and black pepper to the taste

- Four tablespoons coconut cream

Directions:

In a bowl, mix cream with turmeric, ginger, salt and pepper, whisk, add chicken pieces, toss them well and leave aside for 2 hours.Transfer chicken to your preheated air fryer, cook at 370 degrees F for 25 minutes andserve with a side salad.

36. Chinese Chicken Wings

- 16 chicken wings Two tablespoons honey

- Two tablespoons soy sauce

- Salt and black pepper to the taste

- ¼ teaspoon white pepper

- Three tablespoons lime juice Directions:

In a bowl, mix honey with soy sauce, salt, black and white pepper and lime juice, whisk well, add chicken pieces, toss to coat and keep in the fridge for 2 hours. Transfer chicken to your air fryer, cook at 370 degrees F for 6 minutes on each side, increase heat to 400 degrees F and cook for 3 minutes more.

Beef and Pork Recipes

37.   Beef Curry

- 2 pounds beef steak, cubed

- Two tablespoons olive oil

- Three potatoes, cubed

- One tablespoon wine mustard

- Two and ½ tablespoons curry powder

- Two yellow onions, chopped

- Two garlic cloves, minced

- 10 ounces canned coconut milk

- Two tablespoons tomato sauce

- Salt and black pepper to the taste

Directions:

Heat a pan that fits your air fryer with the oil over medium-high heat, add onions and garlic, Stir and simmer for 4 minutes, then stir well.

Add potatoes and mustard, stir and cook for 1 minute.

Add beef, curry powder, salt, pepper, coconut milk and tomato sauce, stir, cook at 360 degrees F for 40 minutes.

Divide into bowls and serve.

38.   **Beef and Cabbage Mix**

- Two and ½ pounds beef brisket

- 1 cup beef stock

- Two bay leaves

- Three garlic cloves, chopped

- Four carrots, chopped

- One cabbage head, cut into medium wedges

- Salt and black pepper to the taste

- Three turnips, cut into quarters

Directions:

Put beef brisket and stock in a large pan that fits

your air fryer, season beef with salt and pepper, add

garlic and bay leaves, carrots, cabbage, potatoes

and turnips, cook at 360 degrees F and cook for 40 minutes.

Divide among plates and serve.

Vegetable Recipes

39.   Balsamic Artichokes

- Four big artichokes, trimmed

- Salt and black pepper to the taste

- Two tablespoons lemon juice

- ¼ cup extra virgin olive oil

- Two teaspoons balsamic vinegar

- One teaspoon oregano, dried

- Two minced garlic cloves

Directions:

Season the artichokes with salt and pepper, fry them with half the oil and half the lemon juice, place them in the fridge and cook for seven minutes at 360 degrees F.

Meanwhile, combine the remaining lemon juice and vinegar, the remaining oil, salt, pepper, garlic and oregano in a bowl and stir well.

Arrange the artichokes on a tray, drizzle over the balsamic vinaigrette and serve them.

40.   **Cheesy Artichokes**

- 14 ounces canned artichoke hearts

- 8 ounces cream cheese

- 16 ounces parmesan cheese, grated

- 10 ounces spinach

- ½ cup chicken stock

- 8 ounces mozzarella, shredded

- ½ cup sour cream

- Three garlic cloves, minced

- ½ cup mayonnaise

- One teaspoon onion powder

Directions:

Mix artichokes with stock, garlic, spinach, cream

cheese, sour cream, onion powder and mayo, toss,

cook at 350 degrees F for 6 minutes.

Add mozzarella and parmesan, stir well and serve.

Conclusion

An air-fryer is a modern kitchen device used for cooking food instead of using oil by blowing sweltering air around it. It provides a low-fat variant of foods typically fried in a deep fryer. The Air Fryer offers fried foods and meals that are healthier, allowing you to get rid of the carbs that come from fried foods while still offering you the crunchiness, taste, and consistency you like.

CPSIA information can be obtained
at www.ICGtesting.com
Printed in the USA
BVHW061920300321
603711BV00004BA/559